TO Me WITH Love

A DEVOTIONAL ON HEALING, PAMPERING AND LOVING YOURSELF

JUDITH A. CARTER

To Me with Love
A Devotional on Healing, Pampering and Loving Yourself

Copyright © 2018 by Judith Carter

All rights reserved. No part of this publication may be used or reproduced by any means, electronic, mechanical, graphic, including photocopying, recording, taping or by any information storage retrieval system or otherwise be copied for public or private use – other than "fair use" as brief quotations within articles and reviews – without prior written permission of the copyright owner. All definitions, unless otherwise stated are from dictionary.com.

Scripture quotations marked (NIV) are taken from the Holy Bible, New International Version®, NIV®. Copyright © 1973, 1978, 1984, 2011 by Biblica, Inc.™ Used by permission of Zondervan. All rights reserved worldwide. www.zondervan.com

ISBN-13: 978-0-692-14230-1

This book was printed in the United States of America

To order additional copies of this book contact:
LaBoo Publishing Enterprise, LLC
staff@laboopublishing.com
www.laboopublishing.com
808-517-4783

Preface

In this world, where change is constant, the roles of people are many. Oftentimes, women neglect themselves because of taking care of children, spouses, pets and loved ones. They make sure everyone else has what they need, but don't take the time to invest in themselves. The purpose of this book is to help you look at yourself; acknowledging areas in your life where you may struggle…especially on how to love and forgive yourself, healing yourself and knowing it's okay to pamper yourself (without guilt).

Read the book, then re-read it and apply the principles! Loving yourself enough to heal is the greatest gift you can give yourself. Watch the transformation unravel as you really begin this amazing journey…. the new and improved you is just "a turn of the page" away!

Acknowledgement

I would like to thank God for sustaining me when I felt I had no life left in me and for giving me the ability to recognize the gifts He put inside me. I would like to say thank you to my children (Aubry, Chad and Jordan) for supporting me even though they may not have understood my journey. For being receptive of me having to do what I needed for myself and understanding this was my time to move in the direction God had called me. My struggles were to hopefully make life better; every decision and sacrifice I made was for the three of you.

I would like to thank my family and friends (personal and spiritual) who supported me through my trials, gave me a shoulder to lean on and tissue for the tears. For helping me stand tall when I was broken! I could not have made it this far without you all!

Thank you to my church family and the awesome women that walk righteous before God; not saying they are perfect, but they practice perfecting their steps daily.

As I was writing this book, I realized it was a cleansing process; I experienced every "day" of this book. It's "my" story, but it's also yours.

I began writing this book during a time when my life was in transition and finished when my transition came full circle. I am now in a new phase of life – a time where I've been healed and can live by and appreciate the advice given throughout these pages. I believe this was by design.

Never underestimate or second guess God's abilities and timing!

Day 1
ACKNOWLEDGEMENT

Acknowledgement means "the recognition of the existence or truth of something!"

Other words for acknowledgement: acceptance, affirmation, assertion, compliance, confession, confirmation and allowance.

The first step to loving yourself is to acknowledge where you are. In doing so, you will see what positive adjustments you need to make for yourself, and to rid yourself of all negative people and habits that may be holding you back. Get rid of the clutter – be it mental, physical or spiritual – and free your space. Allow yourself to be vulnerable to yourself! Open yourself up to receive spiritual gifts and healing, blessings, compliments, the friendships and relationships you deserve.

> **Repeat**
> I am beautiful
> I am loved
> I love myself because I am worthy of love

> **Today's Love Lesson to Self**
> Finding my quiet place!

Treat yourself to the wonderful world of aromatherapy. Treat yourself to the wonderful aromas of Pamper Me Pretty's scented candles. Calm your inner space and enjoy your quiet time! It's okay to be by yourself, it allows you to hear from the Lord on His plans for you!

Day 2
SUBMIT

There are many definitions for submit. The definition being used for this devotional is to subject to treatment or influence.

Other words for submit: comply, bow, obey, agree, yield.

After you acknowledge where you are on your journey and identify the areas you want to improve, submit to yourself and the love you have deep within you. Allow it to come forth and shine. Be the beacon of light for all to see and do not feel guilty for loving the person you see. You are not perfect and that is okay; only our Heavenly Father holds that title, so free yourself of the stress of trying to fill those shoes.

> **Repeat**
> I am free to be me
> I am free to love all of me
> I am free

> **Today's Love Lesson to Self**
> Life's Little Pleasures

I will submit to some guilty pleasures of pampering myself. Today I will take a hot soak bath using Pamper Me Pretty's scented "bath teas" to make my bath time more luxurious. I will enjoy the aroma while the oils and salts soften my skin and soothe my muscles.

Day 3
WAKENING

Wakening means "to rouse from sleep; to rouse from inactivity, stir up or excite, arouse, awaken."

Other words for wakening: arise, come to, be roused, get up, open one's eyes, bring to life.

My inner self will be allowed to awaken – get up, come to and be aroused! I will bring to life my inner man to bring life to myself. I will no longer be in bondage to the people, places or things of this world, but instead enjoy all the blessings before me. I will look at life through new eyes and with a positive mind, because I am worth it!

> **Repeat**
> I can see clearly now
> I see me changing
> I accept the change

> **Life's Lesson to Me**
> Seeing Through New Eyes

Because I welcome the awakening within me, I will feed my skin with nourishments from the natural and organic ingredients of Pamper Me Pretty's body butters. My skin will be kissed with its silkiness and softening minerals. I will love hugging me!

Day 4
CONTENTMENT

Contentment means "the state of being contented; satisfaction, ease of mind."

Another word for contentment: happiness

I allow myself to be happy with my decisions and my positive changes. I am okay with saying no, because I don't have to do those things I do not want to do. I will be content with no longer feeling guilty for taking care of me first.

> **Repeat**
> I say yes to my thoughts
> I say yes to my dreams
> I say yes to myself
> And I'm happy about it

> **Today's Love Lesson to Self**
> Dare to Be Free

I will fix my hair in a different style, or maybe I will cut or dye it; either way, I will nourish my hair with Pamper Me Pretty's Epiphany Hair Butter. I dare to do something different today…being carefree is my treat to me!

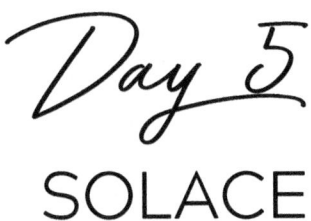

SOLACE

Solace means "something that gives comfort, consolation or relief. To comfort, console or cheer (a person, oneself, the heart, etc.)."

Other words for solace: relief, comfort, cheer and support.

I will allow myself to breathe! Inhale, exhale and repeat slowly. I find comfort in slowing down and taking in every moment life has to offer. What's the old saying, "sit back and smell the roses." Yup, that's what I want to do. I am okay with going slow.

> **Repeat**
> I will not rush the day
> I will not rush myself
> I will take my time
> And I will learn who I am

> **Life's Lesson to Me**
> Roads less traveled… have more scenic views. Enjoy them!

I give me permission to find comfort with my life, to love it until I don't…then I give myself permission to change it to be the way I want it to be. I give myself permission to relax – watching the sunset, feeling the breeze on my skin, drinking some tea. I can do this while curled up reading a book. "In the Still of the Night: A Compilation of My Life in Poetry" is a good book to settle down with as I read beautiful poetry representing different stages of my life.

Day 6
BOLD

Bold means "going beyond the usual limits of conventional thought or action; imaginative. Not hesitating or fearful, to break the rules; necessitating courage and daring; challenging."

Other words for bold: adventurous, forward, fearless, unafraid, courageous, heroic.

I take control of me! I give myself permission to do the things I want to do when I want to and not feel guilty about it. It is okay to put me first and be as daring and adventurous as I would like. Living life day to day, one moment at a time and as if it's my last! I move forward like a lioness protecting her cubs…quiet, stealth, confidence and with strength.

> **Repeat**
> I am not afraid
> So, I will go for it
> And I will do it now

> **Life's Love Lesson to Me**
> Walking out MY Destiny with Eyes Wide Open!

I will take on the world with confidence. I will not be afraid of what's coming my way. I will embrace the challenges, not run from them; and I will be okay if I make a wrong decision along the way (I will not call it a mistake, just not the right choice at that time). I will forgive myself!

I will begin my day with a bold, invigorating shower using an exfoliating sea salt or sugah scrub from Pamper Me Pretty. Scrubbing away the dead weight and dead skin as I take on the world.

Day 7
PEACE

Peace means "the freedom of the mind from annoyance, distraction, anxiety, an obsession etc.; tranquility; serenity."

Other words for peace: calm, quiet and soothing.

It's time to bring calmness to my surroundings, my home and my mind. Quiet the inner and outer noise! Invite the Holy Spirit into your space, giving Him permission to usher in His tranquility and change your atmosphere.

> **Repeat**
> Quiet my mind Lord
> And allow me to hear your voice

> **Life's Love Lesson to Me**
> Loving the Loudness of Being Quiet

I will open the windows and let the breeze blow through. After getting out of the tub/shower, I will lavish my skin with Bath & Body Oil from Pamper Me Pretty and just relax; allowing my spirit to connect with the Holy Spirit as He guides and directs my path. I am at peace!

Day 8
TIRED

Tired means "exhausted, as by exertion; fatigued or sleepy; weary or bored, informal, impatient or disgusted."

Other words for tired: drained, fatigued, sleepy, overtaxed, irritated, broken down, broken-down, empty.

Life can be a challenge. We deal with many relationships – work, personal, spiritual, friendships, educational! There are times when these relationships weigh us down…making us tired. It's at these moments that we must turn our situations over to God, because they are out of our control…however, for those things we can control, we must decide what is best for our spiritual, physical and emotional needs. People who don't want you in their life, respect their decision and find a way to move on; and situations that aren't benefiting you, but are stressing you out or having a negative impact on you, get rid of them. Every decision you make must move you forward toward your goals and destiny. Don't allow life to distract you and tire you out to the point that you are now stagnant!

> **Repeat**
> I am important
> I owe it to myself to rest
> Rest my body, mind and spirit
> I am important!

> **Life's Love Lesson to Me**
> Finding Comfort in Being Still

When tired from worry, work, relationships, school, relax in a hot bath. Use one of Pamper Me Pretty's Bath Bombs (fizzy). They come in a variety of scents, but to help you relax, choose either lavender or chamomile. Allow the oils, and the combination of salts (including Epson) to melt away your tired feelings and enjoy the moment. You deserve it!

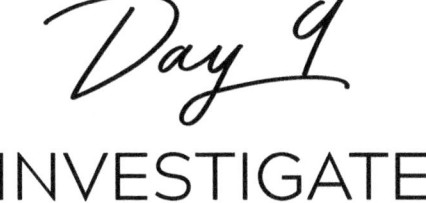

INVESTIGATE

Investigate means "to carry out research or study into to discover facts or information; make a check to find out something; or to observe or study by close examination and systematic inquiry."

Other words for investigate: inquire into, look into, probe, explore, scrutinize, conduct an investigation into, conduct an enquiry into, make inquiries about.

My people are destroyed for lack of knowledge …Hosea 4:6! Love yourself enough to be informed…regardless of what area of life…be it a job, people you bring into your circle, education, community or even the food, drink and products you put in/on your body. Know your ingredients. What you don't know can kill you!

Stay away from the following ingredients in your beauty care products, especially your hair dyes. They have been known to cause cancer.

Hydroquinone, ethanolamine, aminophenol, 2, 4-diaminophenoxyethanol, Phenylenediamine

Other ingredients used in hair dyes that can cause other illnesses such as dermatitis, nausea (if inhaled), and possibly issues with breathing.

Resorcinol, p-phenylenediamne, ammonium hydroxide, sodium metabisulfite toluene, 2-methylresorcinol, nonoxynol-4, nonoxynol-9, phosphoric acid, etidronic acid.

> **Repeat**
> I owe it to me
> To learn all I can
> About what comes in contact with me,
> I owe it to myself
> To be responsible to me!

> **Life's Love Lesson to Me**
> Read, Learn & Live

Know that Pamper Me Pretty's skin and hair care ingredients are quality organic and natural products. They have no preservatives or other artificial ingredients that can be hazardous to your body.

Day 10

ALTERNATIVE

Alternative means "(of one or more things) available as another possibility; offering or expressing a choice; different from the usual or conventional."

Other words for alternative: different, other, another, substitute or replacement.

In life, there is always "another choice that can be applied to almost everything. Alternative lifestyles and changes are the results of conscientious decisions being made. People can choose to have alternative food choices, cleansing products, healthcare items, etc. Example, instead of using fragrant plug-ins…use potpourri around the house. It is a "greener and cleaner" way to scent your atmosphere without inhaling allergenic and/or toxic ingredients.

Invest time into you…because you are worth it! Eat organic and use as many organic products on your skin and in your home as possible. Eliminate processed and sugary foods, eat plenty of fresh fruits and vegetables and whole grains. Eat organic or free-range/cage free eggs and poultry, wild caught fish and drink plenty of water. Exercise, meditate, pray and get plenty of sleep!

> **Repeat**
> It's okay to do things differently
> It's okay to see things differently
> It's okay to be "different"

> **Life's Love Lesson to Me**
> Be Open to Options the Universe Offers You...Think Outside the Box!

Exfoliating Tip

An alternative to bring life to dull looking, uneven or flaky skin is to exfoliate it. Exfoliating is a good way to rejuvenate the skin by sloughing away dead skin cells. Your skin will feel softer and will have a glow! Word of caution….do not use scrubs (exfoliate) if you have any type of inflammation, cuts or scrapes on the skin. Pamper Me Pretty offer a variety of exfoliating products.

Day 11
TIME TO RELAX

Relax means "to release or bring relief from the effects of tension, anxiety, etc.; to become less tense, rigid or firm."

Other words for relax: unwind, calm, take a break, take it easy, sit back, breathe easy.

It is important to find your "me" space and escape from the cares of the day and the world. Relaxing your body, mind and spirit is essential to you being able to continue this journey called life in a healthy manner. Therefore, enjoy a glass of wine, unwind in a hot bath or shower, enjoy some soothing music, watch a movie, read a book, burn a scented candle and get much needed rest!

> **Repeat**
> I must relax
> I can relax
> I will relax

> **Life's Love Lesson to Me**
> Sometimes, NOTHING is the best thing you can do!

Soothing & Relaxing Milk Bath Recipe
- ¼ cup of organic milk powder
- 10 drops of lavender or chamomile essential oil (or your favorite scent)
- 4 drops of jasmine or rose essential oil (or your favorite scent)

Mix essential oils with 6 tablespoons of milk powder. After the essential oil disappears, mix in with the remaining milk powder. When ready to use, add approximately 4 tablespoons to your bath. Soak your body and enjoy!

Day 12
PRAYER

Prayer means "a devout petition to God or an object of worship; a spiritual communion with God or object of worship, as in supplication, thanksgiving, adoration, or confession; a religious observance, either public or private; a petition or entreaty."

Other words for prayer: petition, implore, request help, supplication, plea, appeal, grace, devotion.

Never underestimate the power of prayer. Prayer changes lives, situations and people. There's nothing you can't ask our Heavenly Father in prayer! Be patient with your petitions…some things God will move on quickly, but other times it will be on His time – just know that if you keep a pure heart exercise forgiveness and love, then He will not turn a deaf ear to your requests.

> **Repeat**
> Lord thank you
> I ask you for nothing
> But to offer myself as a vessel
> To use as you will

> **Life's Love Lesson to Me**
> My God's ears are always close to my lips

Pamper Me Pretty has a selection of aromatherapy oils, aerosols and candles just for this occasion…or any occasion you choose. Have them tailor made to your specifications and for your purpose (cleansing, inviting, relaxing, etc.).

Day 13
SELF-PRESERVATION

Self-preservation means "the instinct to act in your own best interest to protect yourself and ensure your survival."

Other words for self-preservation: protection, conservation, self-protection, defense mechanism, survival instinct.

There are many ways a person can infuse self-preservation in their life. Keep negative and toxic people, things and situations out of your life. Learn how to say "no" without guilt, don't overextend yourself, rest and date and treat yourself.

Date yourself! You don't have to wait for someone to take you on a date. Only you know what makes you feel special, so every now and again, it's okay to date yourself!

Treat yourself to the flowers of your choice and put them in a pretty vase…front and center for all to see.

Treat yourself to an outfit, pair of shoes, mani-pedi, hairdressers or a massage. If affordable, do all of them, but if not, pick one!

Treat yourself to breakfast, lunch or dinner...and enjoy

Treat yourself to something sweet...order from your favorite spot and have it delivered to yourself with a little love note to you! (if you have it delivered at work, all would see and you don't have to share who it is from, keep it mysterious...all while smiling on the inside... and out)

Plan an overnight or weekend get-away to your favorite hotel or Bed-n-Breakfast. And order room service!

Repeat
I matter first,
And I owe it to myself to take care of me!

Life's Love Lesson to Me
Don't just survive...Live!

Day 14
ANGRY

Angry means "having a strong feeling of or showing annoyance, displeasure, or hostility; full of anger." "I'm angry that she didn't call me" · "an angry customer" · "Christine had made him angry"

Other words for angry: irate, annoyed, cross, vexed, irritated, exasperated, indignant, aggrieved, irked, piqued, displeased, provoked, galled, resentful, furious, enraged and infuriated.

All that hurt and pain that you've buried, trying to pretend you don't care anymore…those so-called family, friends, Ex's, coworkers, etc. that twisted the knife in your back a little more…yes, go ahead and admit it. You are still angry, and it's okay. Be angry, but in your wrath, do not sin.

It's okay to be angry because anger is a natural emotion…just as hurt, pain, joy, sadness and fear. They are the emotions that drive us to be who we are. Do not deny your emotions, but positively deal with them. Don't let them control you, but you stay in control of them!

Understand that there are stages associated with each emotion, and for you to successfully overcome whatever emotion you are going through, you must go through the stages.

Healthy anger propels you forward or but unhealthy will cripple you and hold you back...especially if you are stuck in it. Admit what made you angry; why it made you angry (or whatever emotion was stimulated); acknowledge if you had a part in it; tell yourself that you are angry....then, ask God to help you deal with your anger; to heal your anger, and then to release your anger so you can move! Accept your feelings and then move forward into a better place...a place of acceptance and peace – only then will you be truly free!

> **Repeat**
> I am angry, Lord
> I need your help
> I accept it
> I release it
> I am healed
> I am free

> **Life's Love Lesson to Me**
> Be angry, then move on!

When you need to wash away your worries, anger, etc. and feel refreshed, use Pamper Me Pretty's Body Bars (soap), in your desired scent, and just lather up a new set of emotions. Not only will you smell wonderful, but your skin will not be dried out from harsh ingredients. Step out of your shower/bath feeling renewed and ready to conquer your day!

Day 15
LONELY

Lonely means "the result of being without the companionship of others, causing or resulting from the state of being alone; isolated, unfrequented, or desolate; without companions; solitary."

Other words for lonely: desolate, reclusive, solitary, down, outcast, alone and companionless.

There comes a time when you must separate yourself from those around you and go on a journey with God…all by yourself. It is during that time that your relationship with Him will become very intimate (if you let Him in). He will show you who you are, but more importantly, He will show you who He is. If open, you will come to a better understanding of your life and the life He wants for you.

God knows your needs! He knows your wants! Just remember that when you feel alone or lonely, that you really are not…for He said, He will never leave you nor forsake you!

> **Repeat**
> Although it may seem nobody
> is here with me,
> Although I might feel alone
> I know I am not
> Because God is with me!

> **Life's Love Lesson to Me**
> God's arms are always wrapped around me!

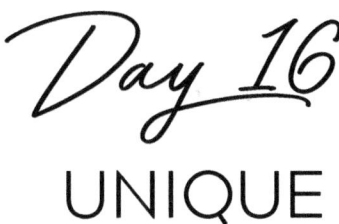

UNIQUE

Unique means "the embodiment of unique characteristics; the only specimen of a given kind; not typical; unusual."

Other words for unique: particular, only, different, exclusive, rare.

I am the only "me" alive. No matter how much one might try to look like me, act like me or talk like me, there will only be one me…one you! I am unique. One of a kind!

> **Repeat**
> There can only be one me
> I am the best me I can ever be
> I am all that God has put in me
> I am undeniably the best me I can be!

> **Life's Love Lesson to Me**
> Being comfortable and confident in my skin

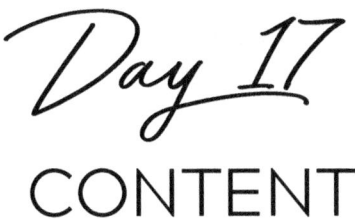

CONTENT

Content means "the state or feeling of being contented; satisfaction; contentment."

Other words for content: fulfilled, comfortable, gratified, at ease, appeased.

When life seems crazy and stressful, remember that there is One who lives deep within you and gives you a sense of peace and contentment. Remember to breathe and be still…not be moved by the chaos that may surround you. Tell yourself it is okay to "sit" and acknowledge the many blessing that surround you…and to be satisfied exactly where you are (not to be confused with being stagnant and non-productive)

Repeat
I choose to be content
I choose to be at peace
I love me enough to be still
And not be moved
By what's going on around me

Life's Love Lesson to Me
I'm exactly where I'm meant to be at this exact time…and I'm ok with that!

Day 18
REJECTION/REJECT

Rejection/Reject means "to rebuff; to deny acceptance, care, love, etc. to (someone); to refuse to take, agree to, accede to, use, believe, etc.; to discard or throw out as worthless, useless, or substandard; cast off or out; to pass over or skip from."

Other words for rejection/reject: turn down, refuse, discard, cast down, discredit, exclude, renounce, pass by.

Everything you do or say will not be accepted by everyone, and you must realize and accept that it's okay. Don't let someone else's rejection of you, your ideas, suggestions and deeds define who you are at that moment. Tell yourself, despite how much it may hurt, that it's okay because everyone is entitled to feel what they want. Just remember to let it be *their* feelings and do not allow it to engulf you and pull you down. I remember God said in Hebrews 13:5 "I will never leave your nor forsake you," so no matter what, I am ok because their rejection does not define who you are!

> **Repeat**
> It's okay that you don't accept me or my ideas
> Your views and rejection of me don't define who I am
> I accept your rejection although I do not agree with it
> I'm okay

> **Life's Love Lesson to Me**
> Others don't define me; I define myself.
> I know who I am and my capabilities...and I love it!

Day 19

"ME" TIME

"Me" time means "time spent relaxing on one's own terms as opposed to working or doing things for others, seen as an opportunity to reduce stress or rest; the time a person has to himself or herself, in which to do something for his or her own enjoyment."

Other words for "me" time: personal time

You owe it to yourself to take care of you! Don't allow everything and everyone else to become the priority in your life. Your life matters! How you take care of yourself will determine just how long you will be around to enjoy life. Quality of life is key!

> **Repeat**
> Sometimes, life is too short to have do-overs
> Sometimes it's not!
> I will not leave it to chance
> Right now, I choose to do what is best for me
> Because it's MY time

> **Life's Love Lesson to Me**
> I'm doing ME!

In this next section, I want to introduce some alternative medicine practices – holistic modalities to consider on your journey of taking care of you. Some services you may be familiar with, while others may seem a bit foreign. Keep an open mind! There is nothing "spooky" about some of these services, as one may have thought.

Holistic services are services that address the "whole" body . . . that's mind, body and spirit! Holistic practitioners believe that to heal the body, they must heal the "whole" person. Usually, when symptoms show up in the mind (mental)…i.e. anger, if left unaddressed, it will manifest in the physical…i.e. skin rashes. So, in holistic practices, the practitioner tries to get to the root of the issues that are causing the physical (or spiritual and mental) issues. Everything is connected!

Now that you have a better understanding, let's begin!

Day 20
MEDITATION

Meditation is a practice where the individual uses techniques (i.e., breathing, prayer, etc.) for relaxing the body and calming the mind.

Other words for meditation: quiet time, reflection, deep thought, pondering, self-examination.

This may seem like an easy act to accomplish, but it is not. It requires discipline and consistency until it becomes a part of your lifestyle. Meditation helps with such ailments as high blood pressure, anxiety, depression, irritable bowel syndrome (IBS) and insomnia.

Meditation increases a person's state of calmness, it is physically and mentally relaxing, it helps improve psychological imbalances, it enables a person to calmly cope with illnesses and it over-all improves a person's health and well-being. Meditation can be done lying down or in a sitting position; in complete quietness or with very soft music. Meditation helps people clear the "clutter" in their mind; therefore, aiding in mental clarity and a sense of being refreshed.

If this is a practice you are familiar with, consider learning more about it and implementing it into your lifestyle. It will help you remain balanced and calm when dealing with everyday issues. It's a good place of escape when tensions have escalated. When the body is calm, the stress hormones automatically released in your body (fight or flight) will not tax your organs, which are damaging over a long period of time.

So, invest a little time in you! Establish a quiet meditation room or space in your home, adorn it with scented candles, pillows, soft music and/or whatever else you need to help you feel comfortable. Let it be your little piece of heaven on earth!

> **Repeat**
> I will practice until I become disciplined
> I will implement change until it becomes permanent
> I will find and achieve my quiet time

> **Life's Love Lesson to Me**
> Whole is my goal... as I quiet my soul!

Pamper Me Pretty has a selection of aromatherapy oils that would be suitable to help set the mood for meditation…helping bring the mind and body into a sense of calm by opening the senses.

Day 21
PRAYER

Prayer is "a religious observance, either public or private, consisting wholly or mainly of prayers."

Other words for prayers: petition, entreaty.

Prayer is very similar to meditation, but it is approached from a spiritual point of view. It is a time to commune with our Heavenly Father.

Just as meditation, you can establish a Prayer Room/Closet/Space that is quiet and comfortable, so you can begin your prayer time. Again, you can burn candles, have scented oils, etc. to usher in the presence of God. Prayer is not to be rushed, and it is not where you go to give God a shopping list of items you want from Him. You must learn how to be still, so you can hear!

Prayer helps with the spiritual piece of living a holistic life. If a person is perplexed in their spirit, that will also manifest into their mental and physical states (i.e. lack of faith makes a person worry, worry turns into anxiety which then begins to impose on sleep and appetite and other digestive issues). Prayer helps a person stay grounded. When you are grounded your body is in a state of homeostasis…. balance! When you feel balanced everything around you will become manageable. After all, you attract what you put out into the atmosphere!

> **Repeat**
> Lord draw me closer to you
> Let me hear your voice
> Bring me to a peaceful state
> While understanding your plan

> **Life's Love Lesson to Me**
> Be still and listen!

Day 22
MASSAGE THERAPY

Massage therapy is "the scientific manipulation of the soft tissues of the body, consisting primarily of manual (hands-on) techniques such as applying fixed or movable pressure, holding, and moving muscles and body tissues."

Other words for massage therapy: rub-down, rubbing, manipulation, kneading, reflexology, shiatsu, acupressure, chiropractic treatment.

Everyone has taken the time out to have a massage performed (and for those of you who haven't, you are missing it). This is a very relaxing technique that you should treat yourself to…self-indulgence… massage is all about you.

Massage stimulates circulation, it relaxes tired muscles and the mind, it can help ease tension and stress…. it's just a wonderful experience. Aren't you worth it!

There are different types of massage. Some are listed below…choose the best fit for you. Always make sure your massage therapist is licensed in your state and has the appropriate experience and skills to perform the appropriate massage.

Swedish Massage
This is the most popular type of massage. It's light to medium pressure helps alleviate stress, reduce pain, improves one's mood and promotes relaxation.

Deep Tissue Massage
Deep Tissue is like Swedish massage; however, the focus is on the deepest layer of muscles to target knots and release chronic muscle tension. For some people, this can be painful.

Trigger Point
A trigger point is a tight area within muscle tissue that causes pain in other parts of the body. Trigger Point Massage is designed to alleviate the source of the pain through a series of isolated pressure and release.

Sports Massage
For athletes of every kind, this massage is specific to your sport, with concentration on an area of concern (i.e. knee, back or shoulder).

Hot Stone
Hot stone massage dissipates tension, eases muscle stiffness in addition to improving circulation and possibly metabolism. Usually for every 1 ½ -hour session of hot stones used, it will promote deeper muscle relaxation with strategic placement of smooth, water-heated stones, at key points on the body. Therapists can also include a customized massage, with the use of hot stones, for complete and lasting wellness.

Reflexology
Reflexology applies pressure to areas in the hands and feet called "reflex zones." It helps reduce stress, concentrates on conditions of the feet and ankle and increases a person's relaxation.

Cranial Sacral Therapy
Gentle techniques addressing the bones of the head, spinal column and sacrum. It is a good massage technique for those suffering from headaches, back pain, TMJD, and neck pain.

Prenatal Massage
For you expecting moms, this massage is a great choice for prenatal care. It will differ for each person based on the needs and/or requests.

Geriatric Massage
Now this massage might not be for you, but we all have parents we can share this information with. This massage technique relieves anxiety and depression while maintaining and improving the overall health in elderly persons.

> **Repeat**
> There is nothing better than being pampered
> I'm allowing myself to relax and heal through the power of touch

> **Life's Love Lesson to Me**
> Stop procrastinating and/or making excuses...book the massage appointment!

Pamper Me Pretty has massage oils to address headaches, tension, calmness, sinus pain, muscle stiffness and joint pain that would be complementary to any massage session. Let your body be indulged and drink up the goodness of therapeutic massage oils.

Day 23
ACUPUNCTURE

Acupuncture is "a Chinese medical practice or procedure that treats illness or provides local anesthesia by the insertion of needles at specified sites of the body."

Other words for acupuncture: stylostixis

Okay…keep an open mind! You owe it to yourself to learn and appreciate other methods of healing the body, mind and spirit. Acupuncture is a practice used in Traditional Chinese Medicine (TCM). It is a very ancient practice that has been used in China for thousands of years. Western medicine eventually incorporated the use of acupuncture in some of its practices, but it is still viewed as an alternative or complimentary medicine and not recognized as mainstream western medicine. However, it doesn't mean that this practice doesn't work. It does, I can attest to it! You owe it to yourself to achieve optimal health, and sometimes that means stepping out of your comfort zone.

Acupuncture focuses on restoring the imbalance of energy in the body. The general theory of acupuncture is based on the premise that there are patterns of energy flow (what the Chinese refer to as Qi…pronounced Chee) through the body. This energy flow is essential for optimal health. When there's a disruption of this energy flow, it is believed that it's the beginning basis for the development of disease in the body. Acupuncture may correct imbalances of energy flow by inserting hair-like needles at points (called meridians) close to the skin. Again, keep an open mind.

One of the main goals of this practice is to promote and restore balance and energy in the body, which will also promote relief and/or healing for a large array of medical conditions such as: rheumatoid arthritis, anxiety, depression, irritable bowel syndrome (IBS), neurological conditions (migraines, Parkinson's disease), and other painful and chronic conditions.

Please make sure before receiving acupuncture, your practitioner is licensed and skilled to perform these services. Not done properly could cause more harm to the body/person.

Repeat
I will be open to new experiences
I will explore other healing modalities
I believe in my body's ability to heal itself naturally

Life's Love Lesson to Me
Be open to receive what has been organically provided

Day 24
COLON HYDROTHERAPY

Colon hydrotherapy is relating to irrigation of the colon for cleansing purposes; irrigation of the colon by injecting large amounts of fluid high into the colon

Other words for colon hydrotherapy: colonics, colon irrigation

The key is an open mind…I will continue to say that throughout this journey!

This is a topic that may be a little uncomfortable to speak on…not to mention, if you've never experienced a colon cleanse, may seem a bit taboo. This is one of the best ways to show yourself that you really care about you. First, as women, we will go for our mammogram to ensure breast cancer is not going undetected (and for men, prostate screenings). Well, colonics is a way of preventing colon cancer.

If you think about it, we consume so much over our lifetime that becomes impacted in our intestinal tract. Yes, there is a lot that "passes", but not everything. Well this is where the colon cleanse becomes beneficial. Colon cleanses can assist in improving your body's health and wellness, including reducing your risk of colon cancer. Here are some other areas colon cleanses help:

- Improves the effectiveness of the digestive system (getting rid of undigested waste)

- Improves regularity and prevents constipation (constipation causes a sluggish digestive system and releases toxins into the bloodstream)

- Increases energy

- Increases absorption of vitamins and nutrients

- Improves concentration

- Jump starts the weight loss process

- Decreases risk of colon cancer

- Increases fertility (fat is estrogen-based, and if too much is present, becoming pregnant becomes more difficult. A colon that is impacted with years of buildup can bear down on the uterus and surrounding reproductive organs in women, causing strain).

- It helps maintain the body's pH balance in the bloodstream. When the body is too acidic from foods consumed, blockages are formed in the colon. The blockages contribute to colon tissue becoming inflamed and diseased, which in turn hinders the absorption of minerals, vitamins and water into the bloodstream. Unfortunately, when this occurs, the environment is conducive for molds, bacteria, parasites, fungus and fecal material to enter the bloodstream and tissue. Not only will this throw off a person's pH balance, but it will eventually wreak havoc on your body's organ systems.

Colon hydrotherapy improves whole-body well-being

Don't you owe it to yourself to cleanse your colon, so you can promote energy and good health?

Repeat
I will get rid of the junk inside of me
I will feed my body good and organic foods when possible
Because if I take care of my body
My body will take care of me

Life's Love Lesson to Me
What goes in, eventually comes out!

Day 25
EXERCISE

Exercise is "bodily or mental exertion, especially for the sake of training or improvement of health."

Other words for exercise: activity, calisthenics, gymnastics, employment, application, practice, performance, ritual, discipline, drill, school, employ, apply, exert and practice.

There is nothing like moving your body to make it feel better. Contrary to belief, the best thing you can do for an achy, sore and stiff body…is move it! Your body continues to deteriorate when you choose to live a sedentary (inactive) lifestyle. Now of course, all things are to be done in moderation. When you have physical challenges, consult your physician to understand what your limitations are, so you don't impose more injury on yourself.

Exercising helps with blood circulation, insomnia, energy, it helps fight against plaque buildup in the arteries and it gets the body into shape, which ultimately promotes a positive mood and outlook because you feel good about yourself. Some relatively easy movements people can do, regardless of whether they are beginners or not are:

- Stretching
- Walking
- Swimming
- Dancing

The more you move, the better you feel…you will begin to feel more energetic. Almost youthful, (after the soreness disappears). No pain, no gain!

Repeat
Exercise keeps my body in shape
Exercise keeps me moving
Movement keeps me feeling young
I will exercise and move
Even when I don't want to

Life's Love Lesson to Me
I will be the best and most fit me, I can be!

Day 26
MANICURE-PEDICURE

Manicures and pedicures are "a cosmetic treatment of the hands and feet, fingernails and toenails, including trimming and polishing of the nails and removing cuticles."

Other words for manicures and pedicures: mani-pedi.

Do not overlook the importance of pampering your hands and feet. Not only does having the pretty polish and designs make the hands and feet more attractive, but it also renders what should be a very relaxing hand and foot massage.

Hands and feet, especially the feet, go through a lot of daily strain. Picking up, putting down, gripping, releasing, writing, carrying, walking, climbing, running and basically, supporting all your weight. Have you ever stopped to think about how much pressure your feet carry daily…the miles walked daily? Well it's a lot. Make your mani-pedi session a deluxe if the establishment offers it. This will usually consist of paraffin wax treatments/wraps, scrubs to exfoliate the skin, hot towel wraps and extensive hand and foot massages in addition to the regular service.

> **Repeat**
> There is no harm in treating myself
> I owe it to me!

> **Life's Love Lesson to Me**
> Go ahead, live a little…. I owe myself the little "extras" in life!

Pamper Me Pretty is a supplier of Zoya Nail Polishes. They are heavier lacquers that are natural based and do not add the strong additives like formaldehydes (which are harmful) to its products. They also come in a large variety of colors

Day 27
VAGINAL STEAMING

Vaginal steaming is an ancient practice treatment that provides a **steam** 'facial' for the vagina with the goal of detoxing the vagina.

Other words for vaginal steaming: vaginal steam, v-steam, chai-yok or bajos.

Keeping an open mind!

Vaginal steaming is a practice that can be traced back many centuries to many cultures to include, Asian, African, Caribbean, Native American and parts of South America. With this practice, you will sit over an open chair covered by sauna capes that are strategically placed over you. Vaginal steams are to help women increase fertility, soothe menstrual cramps, vaginal and urinary infections, cysts, hemorrhoids and offer other health benefits. Some establishments will have you do a series of stretches and other supporting postures to open the hips, which will help circulation to the womb area, all while removing tension in the back and pelvis areas. Included in your session is usually aromatherapy, which helps opening the chakras/pathways of energy. During this process as you are seated, herbs are heated to release herbal steam directly into the vaginal tissue. This process allows for a full body sweat detox, allowing the steam to be absorbed through the skin through opened pores. You can continue experiencing the detox (mentally, physically, spiritually and emotionally) up to a few days after the vaginal steam. Usually, an herbal formula is provided to you to help support your detox and healing process (mental, physical, spiritual and emotional). It's an awesome experience, and another step to caring for you!

> **Repeat**
> I am open to care for and pamper myself
> From head to toe
> And every private place in between

> **Life's Love Lesson to Me**
> It's okay to be in the "hot seat," if it's benefiting me!

Day 28
DIET

Diet is the "food and drink considered in terms of its qualities, composition, and its effects on health; a particular selection of food, especially as designed or prescribed to improve a person's physical condition or to prevent or treat a disease."

Other words for diet: food, dietary regimen, nourishment

Well, when talking about your diet, we are talking about food/beverage consumption. It is important that you watch refined sugars and processed foods and drinks. Although they may taste good, they are not good for you. Learn how to read and understand labels. A safe rule to follow is – if you can't pronounce it, you don't want to eat it.

Foods should be fresh, organic whenever possible, eaten raw when possible (fruits and veggies), drink plenty of water (not sugary drinks nor drinks full of caffeine), and your food selections should be very colorful and from a large variety. Try to stay away from canned foods (especially fruits and veggies) because they are full of sodium and usually additives, preservatives (to expand shelf life), dyes and other artificial ingredients. The fresher the foods, the more nutrients you get from it.

I am not saying you can't treat yourself to something sweet and yummy every now and again, but don't let it be your norm. Take care of your body by fueling it with good and wholesome foods, and it will take care of you!

Start by making little changes in the diet and continue until you are omitting a lot of the junk foods. Steam, sauté and grill foods as opposed to frying. Begin making changes that will eventually become part of your lifestyle!

> **Repeat**
> I am what I eat

> **Life's Love Lesson to Me**
> Make a deliberate effort to eat to live...
> don't live to eat!

Day 29
SLEEP

Sleep is "a natural temporary state of rest during which an individual becomes physically inactive and unaware of the surrounding environment and many bodily functions; a condition of body and mind which typically recurs for several hours every night, in which the nervous system is relatively inactive, the eyes closed, the postural muscles relaxed, and consciousness practically suspended."

Other words for sleep: nap, doze, rest, drowse, catnap, beauty sleep and snooze.

It's no surprise that your body needs an appropriate amount of sleep! Sleep deprivation leads to many conditions – both mental and physical – that over a period, can become detrimental to your health.

Sleep is a time when the body regenerates itself and goes through its own detoxification process. It rids the body of various toxins, rests the digestive tract, refreshes the mind and gives you energy and clarity to get through your days. When a person lacks sleep (or an appropriate amount of sleep), they become lethargic, slow to respond, have brain fog, a loss or impairment of short term memory, lack concentration, get headaches, susceptible to weight gain, become moody and irritable and can even act like a person under the influence of drugs or alcohol.

Not only the items listed above, your overall appearance becomes dull. So, make sure you go to bed early enough to get about 7-8 hours of sleep daily. They really weren't kidding when they said, "I need my beauty sleep." Turn off the television and let your body unwind and go to sleep. I will see you on the other side of your eyelids. Sweet Dreams!

Repeat
I will allow myself to sleep tonight
It will be an undisturbed sleep
The sleep will be peaceful!

Life's Love Lesson to Me
Dare to dream

Day 30

LAUGH

Laugh means to make the spontaneous sounds and movements of the face and body that are the instinctive expressions of lively amusement and sometimes also of contempt or derision.

Other words for laugh: chuckle, chortle, guffaw, giggle, titter, snicker and cackle.

You owe it to yourself to appreciate the little things and the big things. But what's more important is not to take life so seriously that you forget to laugh. Laughter is good for the soul…it makes a merry (happy) heart. It also improves health!

Laughter is contagious. So, even when things seem to be falling apart around you, take a moment to laugh…it will lift your spirits and make you feel better. Let your smile light up the room. Let people see your smile and let it light up the room when you enter it. What has you smiling?

Repeat
My laughter is contagious
My smile is beautiful
I will let the inner me shine through
And I will see it through my smile

Life's Love Lesson to Me
Don't be so serious all the time - laugh, a lot!

Day 31
GIRL, GET YOUR LIFE!

In conclusion, it is important that you take charge of your life. Incorporating a core team of "players" that will help you stay on track, promote growth (mental, physical and spiritual) and to help you look and feel good about yourself!

As a point of reference, I've outlined some key concepts and various services you can use to help you love and appreciate the person God has designed you to be. Your life should constantly be changing for the better. There's no one right way to do things to improve who you are…but it does begin in the mind. Change your mind, you can change your life!

Don't let your life be a spectator sport but become an active player. Take a few people on the journey with you to give you support and encouragement. Keep a journal to track your progress (or lack thereof). But most importantly, Girl, get your life!

A few items to help you on your journey…customize as you see fit!

A good "small" circle of TRUE friends that will keep you in check

(they'll tell you what you <u>Need</u> to hear and not just what you <u>Want</u> to hear…they will speak the truth and keep it real!)

A good **Church Home/Pastor**

A good **Spiritual Accountability Partner/Advisor**

A good **Business Accountability Partner/Advisor**
   (entrepreneurs or those thinking about owning a business)

A good **Retailer of wholesome Skin & Hair Care Products**
   (i.e. Pamper Me Pretty)

A good **Western Medicine Practitioner** (primary care physician)

A good **Eastern Medicine Practitioner** (acupuncturist, traditional Chinese medicine, herbal medicine, colon hydrotherapy, ionic foot detox, remedies, acupressure, chakra healing)

A good **Naturopath Practitioner**

A good **Life Coach/Fitness Trainer** (sometimes you are lucky enough to find someone who does both…a 2 for 1…. but if not, find each separately)

A good **Massage Therapist**

A good **Hairstylist** (especially if you are natural or transitioning)

A good **Dentist** (and yes, there are holistic dentists)

A good, quality **Mattress** for quality sleep

A designated space for "me" time, meditation and prayer

A steady supply of journals and affirmations, mantras

A supply of aromatherapy

An open mind and willingness to make positive changes to heal, laugh and move forward.

www.ingramcontent.com/pod-product-compliance
Lightning Source LLC
Chambersburg PA
CBHW070102100426
42743CB00012B/2640